THE PEGAN DIET SMOOTHIE

Recipes to help you reverse disease optimize health, longevity, and performance.

By

Kim Cox

THE PEGAN DIET SMOOTHIE

Copyright © 2021, By: *Kim Cox*

ISBN: 978-1-956677-01-0

All Rights Reserved. No part of this publication may be reproduced in any form or by any means, including scanning, photocopying, or otherwise without prior written permission of the copyright holder.

Disclaimer:

The information provided in this book is designed to provide helpful information on the subjects discussed. The publisher and author are not responsible for any specific health or allergy needs that may require medical supervision and are not liable for any damages or negative consequences from any treatment, action, application or preparation, to any person reading or following the information in this book.

THE PEGAN DIET SMOOTHIE

Table of Contents

Delectable Smoothie Recipes 5

    Easy Pumpkin Pie Smoothie (Vegan, Dairy Free, Paleo-Friendly) 5

    MIXED BERRY SMOOTHIE RECIPE (WHOLE30, PALEO, VEGAN) 7

    PALEO GREEN SMOOTHIE 8

    STRAWBERRY BANANA SMOOTHIE BOWL 10

    Healthy Mixed Berry Smoothie (Whole30, Paleo, Vegan) 12

    Paleo blueberry banana chia 14

    Easy berry smoothie recipe 16

    Strawberry banana smoothie bowl (paleo + vegan) 18

    Banana date smoothie bowl 20

    Kid-Friendly Smoothie Bowls (Vegan, Paleo) 22

    Sweet Potato Smoothie (Paleo/Vegan) 24

        Vanilla Cheesecake Paleo Smoothie with Protein {Vegan, No Added Sugar} 26

    CLASSIC GREEN SMARTER SMOOTHIE {KETO, PALEO, VEGAN-OPTION} 28

    Cookie Dough Smoothie (Paleo, Vegan) 30

    Green Protein Smoothie (Vegan + Paleo) 32

THE PEGAN DIET SMOOTHIE

No grains or refined Green Smoothie Bowl: Paleo, Vegan 34

Awakening Matcha Smoothie Bowl Recipe 36

Pineapple Green Smoothie 38

CINNAMON PEANUT BUTTER SMOOTHIE 40

Chocolate Avocado Smoothie 41

Whole30 Cherry Smoothie 43

Paleo Key Lime Pie Smoothie 45

Orange Carrot Smoothie with Ginger 47

Paleo and Vegan 5 Ingredient Pineapple Banana Smoothie . 48

Purple Power Smoothie Bowls (Paleo) 50

Chocolate Avocado Smoothie (paleo, vegan, dairy-free options) 52

Creamy pink smoothie bowl (vegan + paleo + refined sugar-free) 54

Paleo Caribbean Sunset Smoothie 57

Dairy-Free Raspberry Smoothie Bowls 58

VEGAN CHOCOLATE RASPBERRY SMOOTHIE 60

Pumpkin Pie Smoothie (Paleo, Vegan, Dairy-Free) 61

Banana & almond breakfast shake {3-ingredients, paleo, vegan} 63

PINEAPPLE MANGO SMOOTHIE 64

Vegan Detox Green Monster Smoothie 65

THE PEGAN DIET SMOOTHIE

Delectable Smoothie Recipes

Easy Pumpkin Pie Smoothie (Vegan, Dairy Free, Paleo-Friendly)

Ingredients

1 (about 13.5 ounce) can unsweetened coconut milk

1 banana, frozen (or better still regular banana with ½ cup ice)

1 Tablespoon of grass fed collagen powder (omit for vegan)

1 cup of pumpkin puree

1 teaspoon of pumpkin pie spice

3 Tablespoons of maple syrup, to taste (or better still raw honey, or other sweetener, optional)

THE PEGAN DIET SMOOTHIE

Directions:

1. First, add coconut milk to blender, and then add remaining ingredients.
2. After which you blend on HIGH for 1 minute, or until smooth.
3. Then, serve with a sprinkle of cinnamon or whipped cream, if desired.

Notes

You can sub alternate sweeteners including stevia, raw honey, erythritol, etc.

THE PEGAN DIET SMOOTHIE

MIXED BERRY SMOOTHIE RECIPE (WHOLE30, PALEO, VEGAN)

Ingredients

- 1/2-3/4 cup of milk of choice
- 1 frozen banana {optional}
- 1 cup of frozen mixed berries
- 1 tablespoon of chia seeds
- 1-2 tablespoons of cashew butter can substitute for any nut or seed butter of choice

Directions:

First, add all ingredients into the blender and blend until desired consistency. NOTE: for a thicker, ice cream like smoothie, I suggest you blend less. Remember, if smoothie is too thick, add more milk of choice.

Notes

1. For thinner smoothies, I suggest you add more milk as needed
2. This smoothie can be chilled for 30 minutes or so.

THE PEGAN DIET SMOOTHIE

PALEO GREEN SMOOTHIE

This recipe is packed with fiber and naturally sweetened with fresh fruit. Simply blend and enjoy the healthiest green smoothie ever!

Serving: Makes about 600 ml (2 ½ cups)

INGREDIENTS

- 2 cups of curly kale
- 1 medium banana {fresh or frozen}
- 1 tablespoon of chia seeds
- 1 to 1 ¼ cups of ice
- ½ to 1 cup of dairy-free milk from a carton
- 4 cups of baby spinach
- 6 pieces strawberries, {fresh or frozen}
- 2 teaspoons of hemp seeds {it is optional}

Directions:

1. First, place everything in a high speed blender in the order listed in the recipe.
2. After which you blend 1 minute or until creamy smooth. A

THE PEGAN DIET SMOOTHIE

3. Then, add more milk or ice cubes for thinner smoothie.

THE PEGAN DIET SMOOTHIE

STRAWBERRY BANANA SMOOTHIE BOWL

Tip:

This recipe is a simple and sweet treat! It's a healthy Paleo + vegan breakfast or snack made with only a few ingredients and feel free to add whichever toppings your heart desires to customize to your tastes.

INGREDIENTS

Ingredients for the smoothie bowl

    1½ cups of frozen strawberries

    ½ cup of Silk Unsweetened Coconut Milk

    1 banana {frozen}

Ingredients for the toppings

    Fresh strawberries {sliced}

    Chia seeds

    Simple Truth Freeze Dried Strawberries + Bananas

    Fresh bananas {sliced}

THE PEGAN DIET SMOOTHIE

Directions:

1. First, combine frozen strawberries, frozen banana, and coconut milk in a blender (I prefer my Vitamix).
2. After which you puree until completely smooth – the mixture should be thick. A
3. After that, add a touch more liquid if necessary to get it to blend completely smooth.
4. Then, transfer to a bowl and add toppings as desired.
5. Enjoy!

THE PEGAN DIET SMOOTHIE

Healthy Mixed Berry Smoothie (Whole30, Paleo, Vegan)

Tips:

This recipe is a thick, creamy and filling mixed berry breakfast smoothie using just four ingredients and naturally sweetened! Easy, quick and extremely satisfying, this recipe is packed with fiber, protein, and fruit, and is naturally vegan, paleo, gluten free, dairy free and whole30 friendly!

Prep Time 1 minute

Cook Time 2 minutes

Servings 1 smoothie

Ingredients

- 1/2-3/4 cup of milk of choice
- 1 frozen banana {it is optional}
- 1 cup of frozen mixed berries
- 1-2 tablespoons of cashew butter can substitute for any nut or seed butter of choice

THE PEGAN DIET SMOOTHIE

1 tablespoon of chia seeds

Directions:

First, add all ingredients into the blender and blend until desired consistency.

NOTE:

1. For a thicker, ice cream like smoothie, I suggest you blend less.
2. However, if smoothie is too thick, add more milk of choice.
3. Add more milk as needed, For thinner smoothies
4. This smoothie can be chilled for 30 minutes or so, for an even thicker smoothie.

THE PEGAN DIET SMOOTHIE

Paleo blueberry banana chia

Yield: 2 smoothies (about 4 cups)

Tip:

This is a 4-ingredient recipe for antioxidant-rich and refreshing blueberry banana chia smoothies.

INGREDIENTS

- 1 ½ cups unsweetened almond milk {divided}
- 1 ½ cups of frozen blueberries
- 2 tablespoons of chia seeds
- 3 medium bananas {sliced and frozen}

Directions:

1. First, in a small bowl, add chia seeds and ½ cup almond milk.
2. After which you whisk until thoroughly combined.
3. After that, cover and chill in the refrigerator for about 10 minutes.
4. Then, add bananas and remaining 1 cup almond milk to a blender.

THE PEGAN DIET SMOOTHIE

5. At this point, blend until smooth, scraping down the sides of the blender as needed.
6. This is when you add blueberries, blending until smooth.
7. Furthermore, remove the chia seed mixture from the refrigerator—it should have thickened to a gel-like consistency.
8. After that, whisk until well mixed.
9. Then, using a rubber spatula or spoon, scrape the chia seed mixture into the blender.
10. Make sure you blend until smooth.
11. Finally, pour into two cups.
12. Enjoy immediately!

THE PEGAN DIET SMOOTHIE

Easy berry smoothie recipe

Prep Time: 5 mins

Cook Time: 0 mins

Yield: 2 smoothies

Tips:

This recipe is quick & easy berry smoothie is ready in 5 minutes!

It is refreshing, packed with antioxidants and delicious.

INGREDIENTS

Easy Berry Smoothie

- 1 cup of unsweetened almond milk
- 1 cup of frozen blueberries
- 1–2 scoops vegan vanilla protein powder (it is optional)
- 2 medium bananas {sliced and frozen}
- 1 cup of frozen strawberries
- 1 cup of frozen raspberries

THE PEGAN DIET SMOOTHIE

Directions:

1. First, add bananas into a blender or food processor.
2. After which you blend until the bananas become crumbly; add almond milk.
3. After that, blend until smooth and creamy, scraping down the sides of the blender as needed.
4. Then, add blueberries, strawberries, and raspberries. B
5. Furthermore, blend until smooth, again scraping down the sides of the blender as needed.
6. Finally, pour into two cups and enjoy!

THE PEGAN DIET SMOOTHIE

Strawberry banana smoothie bowl (paleo + vegan)

Prep Time: 5 minutes

Yield: 1 bowl

Tips:

1. This recipe is a simple and sweet treat!
2. It's a healthy Paleo + vegan breakfast or snack made with but a few ingredients, and feel free to add whichever toppings your heart desires to customize to your tastes.

INGREDIENTS

FOR THE SMOOTHIE BOWL

1½ cups of frozen strawberries

½ cup of Silk Unsweetened Coconut Milk

1 banana {frozen}

FOR THE TOPPINGS

Fresh strawberries {sliced}

THE PEGAN DIET SMOOTHIE

Simple Truth Freeze Dried Strawberries + Bananas

Chia seeds

Fresh bananas {sliced}

Directions:

1. First, combine frozen strawberries, frozen banana, and coconut milk in a blender (I prefer my Vitamix).
2. After which you puree until completely smooth – the mixture should be thick.
3. Then, add a touch more liquid if necessary to get it to blend completely smooth.
4. Finally, transfer to a bowl and add toppings as desired.
5. Enjoy!

THE PEGAN DIET SMOOTHIE

Banana date smoothie bowl

Prep Time: 5 minutes

Yield: 1 bowl 1x

Tips:

1. This recipe is a creamy and sweet treat that tastes like ice cream but is simple and healthy enough for breakfast thanks to a secret veggie that's snuck in there.
2. However, it is time to make you a bowl of this paleo and vegan banana date goodness on the next warm morning for a refreshing breakfast.

INGREDIENTS

1 banana {frozen}

1 Medjool date {pitted}

1 tablespoon of flax seeds

½ cup of almond milk

½ cup of frozen cauliflower {NOTE: steam before freezing for the best flavor}

1 tablespoon of almond butter

THE PEGAN DIET SMOOTHIE

Optional: ½ teaspoon vanilla extract and/or better still ½ teaspoon cinnamon

Directions:

1. First, combine all of the ingredients in a blender (I prefer my Vitamix).
2. After which you blend until smooth + garnish with freeze-dried bananas, almond butter, flax seeds, berries of choice, and/or whatever other goodness you feel like!

THE PEGAN DIET SMOOTHIE

Kid-Friendly Smoothie Bowls (Vegan, Paleo)

PREP TIME 5 MINUTES

SERVINGS 2

Ingredients

Dragon Fruit Bowl:

- 1 large banana
- 1/2 cup of frozen raspberries or strawberries
- 2 tablespoons of apple juice optional
- 1 frozen packet of pitaya
- 1/3 cup of unsweetened almond or nut milk
- 1 tablespoon of chia seeds

Acai Bowl:

- 1 large banana
- 1 tablespoon of almond butter
- 2-3 tablespoons of apple juice optional

THE PEGAN DIET SMOOTHIE

1 frozen packet of acai

½ cup of frozen strawberries or blueberries

1/2 unsweetened almond milk or better still nut milk

1 tablespoon of hemp seeds

Additional toppings:

1/2 cup of fresh strawberries

1/4 cup of flaked or better still shredded coconut

1 kiwi {sliced}

1/3 cup of fresh blueberries

Directions:

1. First, choose between the dragon fruit or acai smoothie bowl, and place those ingredients into a high powered blender.
2. After which you pulse until smooth.
3. Then, adjust for sweetness by adding in apple juice.
4. Finally, top with fresh fruit, nuts, coconut, seeds, bananas, or even granola.

THE PEGAN DIET SMOOTHIE

Sweet Potato Smoothie (Paleo/Vegan)

Prep Time 5 minutes

Servings 1

Ingredients

1 cup of frozen cauliflower rice (about 100 grams)

½ teaspoon of vanilla extract

¼ teaspoon of nutmeg

1 ½ cups of unsweetened vanilla almond milk (or more or less depending on smoothie thickness preference)

1 small sweet potato baked, cut, and frozen* (about 6.5 ounces/1 ½ cups cubed)

1 tablespoon of almond butter

1/2 tablespoon of cinnamon

1 teaspoon of maple syrup (optional)

Optional additions: collagen, chia seeds, protein powder, yogurt...

THE PEGAN DIET SMOOTHIE

Directions:

1. First, put all ingredients to a Vitamix or high powdered blender and blend until smooth, about 1 minute.
2. Then, top with toppings or drink as it.

Notes

1. Remember, for you to bake sweet potato, preheat oven to 400 degrees and bake from 30-40 minutes until soft and can be pierced with a knife.
2. Then, cut into large cubes and place in the freezer until frozen solid.

THE PEGAN DIET SMOOTHIE

Vanilla Cheesecake Paleo Smoothie with Protein {Vegan, No Added Sugar}

Tip:

1. This amazingly delicious recipe is loaded with good stuff and it's sweetened with dates and is completely paleo, dairy free, and vegan.
2. You can add a scoop of your favorite protein or collagen for a nourishing snack or dessert!

Prep Time: 5 minutes

Servings: 4

Ingredients

4 medjool dates pitted (**NOTE:** softened first, if necessary)

½ cup unsweetened almond milk

2 1/2 Tablespoons of fresh lemon juice about 1 lemon

Crumbled vanilla wafer cookies {it is optional}

2/3 cup of raw cashews {**NOTE:** I did not soak them first but you can if you prefer}

THE PEGAN DIET SMOOTHIE

3/4 cup of full fat coconut milk

2 teaspoons of pure vanilla extract

Handful ice

1 scoop of protein powder or collagen peptides optimal

Directions:

1. First, place all ingredients (except for the cookie crumbles) in a high speed blender and blend until very smooth.
2. Then, serve right away topped with cookie crumbles if desired

Notes

1. Remember, if you use all coconut milk; make sure it's the "light" version since full fat will be too thick.
2. However, using all almond milk will result in a thinner, less creamy smoothie.
3. For vegan cookie crumbles, I suggest you use my n'oatmeal raisin cookie recipe without the raisins!

THE PEGAN DIET SMOOTHIE

CLASSIC GREEN SMARTER SMOOTHIE {KETO, PALEO, VEGAN-OPTION}

Serves: it is one very large serving or two smaller servings

Ingredients

1 very large handful spinach

¼ cup of blueberries (feel free to add a little more if this is serving two)

½ avocado

Sprinkle shredded coconut on top

2 cups of unsweetened almond milk (or better still other non-dairy milk)

1 very large handful frozen zucchini (NOTE: it can also be fresh)

1-2 heaping scoops of vanilla protein (NOTE: two scoops for two servings)

1 tablespoon of chia seeds

THE PEGAN DIET SMOOTHIE

Directions:

1. First, starting with the liquid first, add all of the ingredients to your high speed blender.
2. After which you blend until smooth and creamy.
3. Then, serve topped with your coconut or other crunchies on top!

THE PEGAN DIET SMOOTHIE

Cookie Dough Smoothie (Paleo, Vegan)

Prep Time: 10 minutes

Cook Time: 0 minutes

Yield: serves 1-2 1x

Tip:

This recipe tastes like ice cream, but is healthy, nourishing, and high in protein and contains hidden veggies and it's perfect for any meal of the day!

Ingredients

½ heaping cup frozen cubed sweet potato (about 80g)

2 scoops of vanilla protein powder

Handful chocolate chips

1 heaping cup frozen cauliflower florets (about 125g)

½ ripe banana (about 75g)

1 heaping Tablespoons of almond butter (preferably sunflower seed butter for nut free)

Plant based milk (add 1 Tablespoon at a time, as needed)

THE PEGAN DIET SMOOTHIE

Directions:

1. First, slightly defrost frozen cauliflower and sweet potato by warming in the microwave for 15 seconds.
2. After that, in a food processor or high powered blender, blend cauliflower, sweet potato and banana for a few seconds.
3. After which you stop to scrape the sides, and then blend a few seconds more.
4. Furthermore, add in remaining ingredients (except chocolate chips) and blend until smooth, stopping to scrape the sides every so often.
5. At this point, add more liquid as needed.
6. This is when you add chocolate chips to the smoothie and pulse a few times until combined.
7. Finally, scoop smoothie into a bowl and eat!

THE PEGAN DIET SMOOTHIE

Green Protein Smoothie (Vegan + Paleo)

Yield: 2

Prep time: 6 MINUTES

Tip:

This is one of the healthiest, yet most delicious, green smoothies I've tried!

Ingredients

- 1 cup of spinach
- 1 thumb-sized piece of fresh ginger {peeled}
- 1 heaped tablespoon of hemp protein
- 1 1/2 cups of unsweetened almond milk
- 2 cups of chopped mango
- 2 small green apples, chopped (skins on, core removed)
- 2 tablespoons of chia seeds
- 1 teaspoon of spirulina powder

THE PEGAN DIET SMOOTHIE

Directions:

1. First, add everything to a high-powered blender and mix until smooth. A
2. After which you add some ice cubes if you want to help make it colder and thicker.
3. Then, taste and adjust, if needed. NOTE: if it's too thick, I suggest you add more almond milk.
4. Finally, pour into two large glasses.
5. Serve and enjoy!

Notes

However, if you're unsure of the taste of spirulina, as it can be quite strong, start with 1/2 teaspoon and work your way up. Feel free to add up to a tablespoon!

THE PEGAN DIET SMOOTHIE

No grains or refined Green Smoothie Bowl: Paleo, Vegan

Tips:

This Delicious recipe is great to start a day with its goodness of spinach, banana, green grapes, and mango, avocado and almond milk.

Prep Time 5 mins

Servings: 1

Ingredients

- 1 banana
- ¼ cup of unsweetened almond milk
- ½ cup of green grapes
- 1 ½ cup of spinach {packed}
- ½ cup of chopped mango {or small mango}
- ½ avocado

Topping

Blueberries

THE PEGAN DIET SMOOTHIE

Hempseeds

Banana

Mango

Directions:

1. First, in a blender or food processor process all ingredients for smoothie bowl into fine consistency and transfer to a bowl and top with toppings.
2. Enjoy.

THE PEGAN DIET SMOOTHIE

Awakening Matcha Smoothie Bowl Recipe

Tip:

This refreshing recipe fuses super foods match a, chia and pomegranate for a satisfying and healthy, how to best kick start your day.

Ingredients

- 2 cups of unsweetened almond milk
- 1/2 cup of unsweetened coconut flakes
- 1 Tablespoon of chia seeds
- 3 large frozen bananas {sliced into chunks}
- 2 Tablespoons of match a green tea powder
- 1/2 cup of raspberries
- 1/2 cup of pomegranate arils

Directions:

1. First, place almond milk, frozen banana, and match a powder in a blender.
2. After which you blend on high until smooth.
3. Then, divide smoothie between two bowls.

THE PEGAN DIET SMOOTHIE

4. Finally, top each bowl with pomegranate arils, raspberries, chia seeds and coconut flakes or toppings of your choice.
5. Enjoy right away.

THE PEGAN DIET SMOOTHIE

Pineapple Green Smoothie

Prep Time: 5 minutes

Cook Time: 0 minutes

Yield: 1 smoothie 1x

Tips:

This recipe is made with only 5 ingredients! I

However, it's packed with minerals, vitamins, antioxidants and will help keep you full and hydrated between meals.

Ingredients

- 1 cup of baby spinach leaves
- 1 Tablespoon of hemp hearts
- 1 cup of unsweetened full fat coconut milk
- 1 cup of frozen pineapple (feel free to use fresh in the same quantity but won't end up with a cold smoothie)
- 1 pitted medjool date

THE PEGAN DIET SMOOTHIE

Directions:

1. First, blend all ingredients in a high speed blender until smooth.
2. Then pour, drink and enjoy!

THE PEGAN DIET SMOOTHIE

CINNAMON PEANUT BUTTER SMOOTHIE
INGREDIENTS

1/3 cup of almond butter, or better still organic peanut butter, if you want

1 cup of milk of choice (I prefer to use my homemade coconut milk)

2 cups of ice

2-3 ripe bananas

1/2 cup of applesauce (it is optional)

1 tablespoon of chia seeds

1 teaspoon of cinnamon

Directions:

First, combine all ingredients in blender and blend on high until smooth

THE PEGAN DIET SMOOTHIE

Chocolate Avocado Smoothie

Tips:

This recipe tastes like a rich chocolate milkshake, while being dairy-free and naturally sweetened with fruit.

PREP TIME 5 minutes

SERVINGS 1

INGREDIENTS

- 4 Medjool dates {pitted}
- 1 heaping tablespoons of cacao powder
- 1 heaping cup of ice cubes
- 3/4 cup of water
- ¼ avocado
- ½ teaspoon of vanilla extract
- 1 handful fresh baby spinach (it is optional)

Directions:

1. First, in a high-speed blender, combine the dates, water, cacao powder, avocado,

THE PEGAN DIET SMOOTHIE

vanilla, and spinach, if using, and blend until very smooth.
2. After which you taste the pudding-like mixture to make sure there's enough sweetness and chocolate flavor to your liking, and adjust anything to your taste. (**NOTE:** Keep in mind that the flavor will be diluted a bit more once you add the ice.)
3. After that, add the ice and blend again, until the smoothie has more of a milkshake-like texture. Remember, you can add as much ice as needed to achieve the texture you want, but keep in mind that extra ice will dilute the chocolate flavor.
4. Then, serve right away.

THE PEGAN DIET SMOOTHIE

Whole30 Cherry Smoothie

Tips:

This protein powder and banana-free makes a healthy snack or delicious treat.

Prep Time 5 minutes

Cook Time 0 minutes

Servings 2 small

Ingredients

- 3 ice cubes
- 1 tablespoon of Chia Seeds
- 1 tablespoon of cashew butter
- 1/4 teaspoon of chlorella powder optional
- ½ cup of water
- 3/4 cup of frozen cherries
- 2 tablespoons of cacao powder
- 2 tablespoon of maple syrup
- 2 dates
- ½ cup of almond milk

THE PEGAN DIET SMOOTHIE

Directions:

1. First, in a powerful blender add the cherries and ice cubes.
2. After which you pulse slightly to chop.
3. After that, add in the remaining ingredients.
4. Then, pour the almond milk and water on top.
5. Finally, blend until smooth.

THE PEGAN DIET SMOOTHIE

Paleo Key Lime Pie Smoothie

Prep Time 5 minutes

Servings 2

Ingredients

¼ cup of macadamia nuts OR better still raw cashews (more carbs), soaked if you do not have a high power blender to pulverize

1/2 medium avocado

1 tablespoon of erythritol or any favorite low carb sweetener to taste, or better still honey, or a banana (last 2 NOT keto)

2 tablespoons of collagen {this is the brand I use, use tessa10 for 10% any order}

Zest of one lime

2 cups of coconut milk {I prefer Trader Joe's Coconut Milk, unsweetened. Feel free to add some of my favorite canned milk variety for extra healthy fats too!}

4 tablespoons of lime juice

Two handfuls of spinach or any greens. {NOTE: I also sometimes add a handful of raw cauliflower}.

THE PEGAN DIET SMOOTHIE

2 tablespoons of coconut butter I use my homemade,

Splash vanilla extract optional

Directions:

First, place all ingredients into a blender and whir until smooth and creamy.

THE PEGAN DIET SMOOTHIE

Orange Carrot Smoothie with Ginger

SERVES: 1

PREP: 5 minutes

INGREDIENTS

- 3/4 Cup of Orange juice
- Honey (it is Optional and to taste)
- 1 Cup of Ice cubes
- 1/3 Cup of Carrot {sliced}
- 1 teaspoon of Fresh ginger {minced}

Direction:

First, place all ingredients into a high-powered blender and blend until smooth!

THE PEGAN DIET SMOOTHIE

Paleo and Vegan 5 Ingredient Pineapple Banana Smoothie

Prep time 5 mins

Serves: 2½ cups

Ingredients

1 large banana {peeled and sliced}

1 – 2 tablespoons of pure maple syrup (feel free to sub raw honey, but honey isn't vegan)

¼ - ½ teaspoon of organic ground ginger (it is optional) (you can also use cinnamon, preferably Ceylon cinnamon)

1 cup of fresh pineapple chunks

1 ½ cups of unsweetened vanilla almond milk (feel free to sub another non-diary milk of choice)

¼ teaspoon of pure vanilla extract

Directions:

1. First, in a large high-speed food processor or blender, add all the ingredients.

THE PEGAN DIET SMOOTHIE

2. After that, blend until it's smooth and creamy.
3. Then, serve and enjoy!

THE PEGAN DIET SMOOTHIE

Purple Power Smoothie Bowls (Paleo)

Prep Time: 15 minutes

Total Time: 15 minutes

Servings: 2 servings

Ingredients

- 1 cup of frozen blueberries
- ½ cup of blackberries
- ½ medium banana fresh or frozen
- 2 ounces protein powder of choice, vanilla or better still chocolate optional
- 1 cup of beets, peeled and diced
- 1 cup of frozen raspberries plus more for topping
- 1 cup of carton coconut milk
- 1/2 medium avocado {skin and pit removed}
- 1 Tablespoon of pure maple syrup

Toppings:

Coconut milk

THE PEGAN DIET SMOOTHIE

Unsweetened shredded coconut

Rolled oats or granola

Additional raspberries, blueberries, or blackberries

Directions:

1. First, in a blender, combine all the ingredients and blend until smooth.

NOTE: for an extra thick smoothie bowl and for additional protein, I suggest you add a scoop of protein powder to this smoothie bowl if you like.

2. After that, add the protein powder and blend again.
3. Then, pour into 2 bowls and top with your choice of toppings.
4. Make sure you serve immediately.
5. Enjoy!

Notes

1. Feel free to use either cooked beets or raw beets.
2. Remember, for a creamier smoothie bowl, use cooked beets

THE PEGAN DIET SMOOTHIE

Chocolate Avocado Smoothie (paleo, vegan, dairy-free options)

Prep Time: 3 min

Cook Time: 0 min

Yield: 1 large smoothie

Ingredients

2 tablespoons of Dutch-process cocoa powder

¼ cup of plain Greek yogurt or coconut cream for the paleo / vegan option

1/2 teaspoon of vanilla extract

85 grams cold avocado flesh (about ~ 1/2 Hass avocado)

1 medium cold banana (NOTE: mine was 120 grams without the peel)

2-4 tablespoons of milk, optional (NOTE: for vegan, dairy-free, or paleo - use non-dairy milk)

Directions

THE PEGAN DIET SMOOTHIE

1. First, blend everything together in a food processor (or better still a blender if you have a very good one - mine requires too much liquid for a thick smoothie like this) until it's very creamy.
2. After which you add more milk until it's the desired thickness.
3. Then, serve immediately or keep covered in the refrigerator for up to one day.

Notes

However, coconut cream (from a can of refrigerated canned coconut milk) or better still coconut milk yogurt will yield a thick smoothie but you could also use coconut milk for a thinner version.

THE PEGAN DIET SMOOTHIE

Creamy pink smoothie bowl (vegan + paleo + refined sugar-free)

Prep Time: 7

Total Time: 7

Yield: 1-2 1x

Tips:

1. However, this vegan smoothie bowl is sweet, tart and super thick. I
2. Remember, that it has fun toppings that compliment the flavors of the nutritious smoothie base; the base is mainly raspberries and bananas.
3. In addition, the raspberries offer dietary fiber, vitamin C and the bananas are a good source of vitamin C, vitamin B6 and fiber.

INGREDIENTS

1 teaspoon of vanilla extract

2 frozen sliced bananas

1/2 cup of unsweetened, plain plant-based milk (I recommend almond milk)

THE PEGAN DIET SMOOTHIE

4 large pitted Medjool dates (or better still substitute 2 tablespoons pure maple syrup)

1/4 cup of blanched and slivered almonds or raw cashews

1 cup of frozen raspberries

Boost it with: 1 tablespoon of chia seeds, hemp seeds and/or ground flaxseed

Toppings:

Raw chunky almond butter (I prefer Trader Joe's brand)

Unsweetened shredded coconut

Raspberry chia jam

Dragon fruit (pitaya), thinly sliced and cut into stars with vegetable cutters

Frozen berries

Directions:

1. First, in a high speed blender, add all the ingredients except the frozen raspberries.
2. After which you blend until smooth and creamy.
3. After that, add the frozen raspberries and blend again until no chunks remain.

THE PEGAN DIET SMOOTHIE

4. Then, taste and adjust sweetness and flavors as desired. P
5. Finally, pour into 1-2 shallow bowls and garnish as shown in the picture. Or, be creative and do your own thing.

NOTES

Note: however, if you need to use more milk to get the blender going try adding only a little bit at a time and if you use too much the smoothie bowl will lose its creaminess and thickness.

THE PEGAN DIET SMOOTHIE

Paleo Caribbean Sunset Smoothie

Tips:

This recipe will make you feel like you're in the tropics.

It is a light, delicious and nutritious all natural drink!

Serves: 24 ounces

Ingredients

>1 cup of frozen strawberries

>1 ½ cups of orange juice {preferably freshly squeezed}

>1 frozen banana

>1 cup of ripe papaya

Directions:

First, place all ingredients in blender and blend on high until smooth.

Notes: things you will need

>**Measuring cups**

>**High-speed blender**

THE PEGAN DIET SMOOTHIE

Dairy-Free Raspberry Smoothie Bowls

Prep time 5 mins

Total time 5 mins

Serves: 2 servings

Ingredients

2 cups of frozen raspberries

1 tablespoon of chia seeds

Raspberry Smoothie Bowl

1 large frozen banana

⅔ Cup of lite canned coconut milk, plus additional if needed

Optional Toppings

Shredded coconut

Chopped hazelnuts

Edible flowers

Fresh raspberries

Shaved dark chocolate

Chia seeds

THE PEGAN DIET SMOOTHIE

Directions:

1. First, in a blender, puree the banana, raspberries, coconut milk, and chia seeds until smooth. NOTE: the mixture will be very thick. S
2. This is when you stop and push down the ingredients, as needed, and if necessary, add more coconut milk.
3. Then, scrape the smoothie into two bowls, and garnish with any or all of the optional toppings, as desired.

THE PEGAN DIET SMOOTHIE

VEGAN CHOCOLATE RASPBERRY SMOOTHIE

PREP TIME 5 minutes

TOTAL TIME 5 minutes

INGREDIENTS

- 1 cup of fresh papaya and raspberry
- 1 tablespoon of cacao powder
- 1 cup of Cauliflower (Steamed then Frozen)
- 1 tablespoon of chia seeds
- 1/2 cup of nut milk

Directions:

1. First, blend everything together
2. Then, add toppings of your choice: I like coconut flakes, granola, cacao nibs, berries

NOTES

However, if you soak chia seeds in the nut milk first for 5-10 min (it turns into chia pudding), then you blend everything else in, the smoothie will turn out creamier.

THE PEGAN DIET SMOOTHIE

Pumpkin Pie Smoothie (Paleo, Vegan, Dairy-Free)

PREP TIME 5 minutes

Ingredients

1 (about 13.5 ounce) can unsweetened coconut milk

1 banana, frozen (or better still regular banana with ½ cup ice)

1 Tablespoon grass fed collagen powder (omit for vegan)

1 cup of pumpkin puree

1 teaspoon of pumpkin pie spice

3 Tablespoons of maple syrup, to taste (or better still raw honey, or other sweetener, it is optional) *

Directions:

1. First, add coconut milk to blender, after which you add remaining ingredients.
2. After that, blend on HIGH for 1 minute, or until smooth.
3. Then, serve with a sprinkle of cinnamon or whipped cream, if desired.

THE PEGAN DIET SMOOTHIE

Notes

You can sub alternate sweeteners including stevia, raw honey, erythritol, etc.

THE PEGAN DIET SMOOTHIE

Banana & almond breakfast shake {3-ingredients, paleo, vegan}

INGREDIENTS

8 whole almonds

1–1/2 medium-large, ripe bananas {frozen}

2/3 cup of nondairy milk (I prefer almond milk)

Optional: large pinch of ground cinnamon

Directions:

1. First, cut the frozen banana into pieces. A
2. After which you add all of the ingredients to a blender and blend until thick and smooth.
3. Serve immediately.

THE PEGAN DIET SMOOTHIE

PINEAPPLE MANGO SMOOTHIE

Prep Time: 10 mins

Cook Time: 5 mins

Yield: 2 servings 1x

INGREDIENTS

1/2 cup of almond milk (or better still other milk of your choosing)

1 cup of frozen pineapple chunks

3 tablespoons of agave nectar (vegan) or better still 100% pure honey (paleo), optional

1/2 cup of ice cubes

1 mango {peeled and sliced}

3 mandarin oranges {peeled}

Directions:

1. First, add ingredients to blender in the order listed.
2. After which you blend on medium to high speed until smooth.
3. Then, top with fresh fruit, chia seeds, or leave as is.

THE PEGAN DIET SMOOTHIE

Vegan Detox Green Monster Smoothie

PREP TIME 5 MINUTES

TOTAL TIME 5 MINUTES

SERVES 1

Ingredients

- 1/2 cup of cucumber {peeled and sliced}
- 1 cup of vanilla almond milk (or alternate milk)
- Large handful of spinach
- ¾ cup of frozen strawberries.
- 1 large frozen banana {broken into pieces}
- 1 ½ cups kale, loosely packed, stems removed (you can also use spinach)

Directions:

1. First, add the almond milk to a high-power blender and toss the banana pieces and kale in; blend on high.
2. After which you add the strawberries and cucumber.
3. After that, blend again until smooth.

THE PEGAN DIET SMOOTHIE

4. Then, add in more almond milk and/or ice for desired consistency.

www.ingramcontent.com/pod-product-compliance
Lightning Source LLC
Chambersburg PA
CBHW071408070526
44578CB00002B/522